Ageless vitality

A guide to a healthy and happy aging experience

John S. Wilkins

Table of contents

Introduction

Having knowledge of the aging process

The process of aging is how the body and its functions get worse with time. Our bodies are less able to repair DNA damage as we age, which results in slower cell division and DNA damage. As a result, physical and cognitive functions deteriorate, and the risk of illness and mortality rises. The "free radical theory," which contends that the accumulation of free radical damage to our cells and DNA is what causes aging, is the most widely recognized view regarding the origins of aging. Inflammation, hormone imbalances, and lifestyle decisions like diet and exercise are other elements that can speed up aging. It has been demonstrated that some therapies, including calorie restriction, exercise, and some medications, can reduce the aging process.

The aging process can also be influenced by hereditary factors. Researchers have uncovered genetic variants that can either raise or decrease a person's risk of developing age-related disorders. They have also identified specific genes that appear to have a role in aging. A good diet and regular exercise have both been linked to a slowed aging process and a lower risk of developing age-related disorders, according to studies.

The cognitive deterioration that frequently takes place as we age is another significant feature of aging. Memory loss, trouble understanding problems, and changes in thinking and reasoning skills are just a few examples of this. Research has proven that there are things we can do to maintain our brains healthy as we age and that cognitive decline is not a necessary aspect of aging.

How essential it is to maintain a healthy lifestyle

The importance of maintaining a healthy lifestyle cannot be overstated because it can improve both physical and mental health. A healthy lifestyle can aid in the prevention of chronic conditions including cancer, diabetes, and heart disease as well as the enhancement of mood, cognitive function, and quality of life.

Regular physical activity is one of the key elements of a healthy lifestyle. Exercise can aid with stress and anxiety reduction, cardiovascular health, muscle strength, and flexibility. The American Heart Association advises engaging in muscle-strengthening activities at least twice weekly in addition to 150 minutes of moderate-intensity aerobic activity or 75 minutes of vigorous-intensity aerobic activity per week.

Maintaining excellent health also requires a balanced diet. Consuming a diet high in fruits, vegetables, whole grains, lean meats, and healthy fats can assist to meet the body's nutritional requirements and lower the risk of developing chronic diseases. Limiting the consumption of added sugars, saturated and trans fats, as well as alcohol, is also vital.

A healthy lifestyle also includes controlling stress, getting enough sleep, abstaining from smoking, and drinking too much alcohol. It might be difficult to maintain a healthy lifestyle, but it can be done gradually and sustainably by making tiny modifications to one's diet, exercise routine, and other behaviors.

Regular doctor's visits are also essential in order to maintain your health and catch any problems early. We may enhance our quality of life, avoid chronic diseases, and live longer, healthier lives by making efforts to maintain a healthy lifestyle.

Maintaining a healthy lifestyle is crucial for older individuals because as we become older, our bodies become less capable of healing and regenerating. We may encounter decreases in physical and cognitive performance as we age, as well as an increased risk of age-related chronic disorders like heart disease, diabetes, and cancer.

For older adults, exercise is especially crucial since it keeps their muscles strong, mobile, and balanced. Regular exercise can also assist to enhance cardiovascular health and lower the chance of falling. Older adults may need to adjust their exercise program, though, to take into account any physical restrictions or long-term medical concerns. A balanced diet is also crucial because they may have unique dietary requirements associated with aging, such as sufficient protein intake to maintain muscle mass and sufficient vitamin and mineral intake to promote bone health. They might also need to be careful about how many calories they consume because their metabolism might be slower than it was when they were younger.

It's crucial for older adults to practice excellent sleep hygiene, control their stress, abstain from smoking, and limit their alcohol intake. The detection and management of any age-related health disorders can also be aided by routine checkups with a healthcare professional.

Additionally, preserving social relationships and keeping the mind active through pursuits like reading, crossword puzzles, and interacting with friends and family might aid in maintaining mental acuity and preventing cognitive decline. Overall, older persons can enhance their quality of life, avoid chronic illnesses, and live longer, healthier lives by making efforts to maintain a healthy lifestyle.

Chapter 1

Longevity Nutrition

Effects of diet on aging

Aging is accelerated by a bad diet that is high in calories, trans fats, and saturated fats. A diet high in nutrients, packed with fiber, and low in calories, on the other hand, can decrease the rate of aging. A good diet can make you up to twenty-seven years younger in real age than a bad one (physiologic age). Poor dietary choices can age you up to 14 years more than the average American, while healthy eating can make you 13 years younger. If you enjoy eating, who doesn't? — discover how to enjoy delicious foods that offer you energy

Overall health is influenced by nutrition, especially in older people. Malnutrition is linked to a faster aging process. In fact, eating a good diet consistently is recognized as one of the key factors in healthy aging.

In addition to the process of food intake, healthy eating habits and optimal nutrition also take into account the absorption, digestion, biosynthesis, catabolism, and excretion of food. Due to oral health issues, difficulty chewing, dry mouth, and diminished appetite, the elderly have a tendency to have more difficulty digesting and absorbing food. This raises their risk of malnutrition.

Anemia, frailty, and blindness are some of the disorders associated with vitamin deficiencies that can result from inadequate food consumption. Osteoporosis, cardiovascular disease, and diabetes are chronic disorders linked to aging. Studies have shown that due to oral health issues or tooth loss, elderly people consume more carbs and less nutrient-rich foods (such as fruits and vegetables). You have a higher risk of developing diabetes and other comorbidities if you consume too many carbohydrates. unchecked oxidative stress can hasten the aging process if the elderly consume a diet low in foods that are nutrient-rich and have antioxidant properties. Vitamins C and E should be consumed in sufficient amounts because they interact with free radicals and stop their development. Additionally, aging is linked to changes in gene expression. These genes are well recognized to play a role in food absorption and nutrient signaling pathways. The elderly may have less stomach acid, which could result in inadequate absorption of calcium, magnesium, iron, and vitamin B12.

vitamins and minerals you need in your diet and how to get more of them:

Iron

Age increases a person's vulnerability to iron deficiency anemia. Iron can support digestive functions, the immune system, and body temperature regulation while also maintaining overall energy levels.

sources of food include spinach, sweet potatoes, asparagus, tomatoes, beets, kale, grains, pork, chicken, fish, eggs, and fowl.

Magnesium

Contains a number of antioxidant qualities and participates in the immunological response, protein synthesis, nerve and muscle function, and blood pressure regulation.

Almonds, spinach, whole grains, cashews, peanuts, fortified morning cereals, black beans, peanut butter, avocado, dark chocolate, brown rice, plain yogurt, banana, kidney beans, salmon, chicken, broccoli, apples, and tofu are some examples of food sources.

Zinc

is necessary for appropriate taste, smell, protein synthesis, immunological function, wound healing, growth, and development. It also plays a variety of roles in cellular metabolism.

Food sources include cashews, chickpeas, yogurt, milk products, whole grains, ready-to-eat breakfast cereals (enriched with zinc), oysters, red meat, chicken, shellfish, eggs, legumes (beans and peas), almonds, and pumpkin seeds.

Selenium

essential for the thyroid and immunological systems
Eggs, brown rice, mushrooms, grains, dairy products, nuts, seeds, fish, seafood, meat, poultry, and spinach are all examples of food sources.

Manganese (Mn)

Alzheimer's disease (AD) and mild cognitive impairment have been linked to low Mn (MCI)
sources of food include quinoa, oats, brown rice, wheat, barley, rye, and garlic.
Iodine is involved in a variety of neural processes.
Fish, shellfish, cereals, eggs, meat, poultry, fruits, vegetables, dairy products, and lima beans are all examples of food sources.

Calcium

Important for bone health since osteoporosis in the elderly increases the risk of falls

Greek yogurt (high in protein and calcium), cheese, cottage cheese, green vegetables (like kale), almonds, oranges, and salmon are among food sources.

Food sources: mushrooms, salmon, tuna, beef liver, cheese, egg yolks, fortified vitamin D milk, or almond milk, which helps the body absorb calcium and is essential for elderly people.

Most individuals need to take vitamin D supplements since they get less sun exposure in the Northern Hemisphere and few items in typical diets to provide enough vitamin D. check your vitamin D levels and consult your physician

Vitamin B

The absorption of vitamin B12 may be hampered by low stomach acid. To prevent or lessen the severity of diseases, B vitamins are required.

Food sources include whole grains, dairy products, meat, fish, poultry, eggs, fortified cereals, spinach, and oranges.

Vitamin C

is well known for its role in protein synthesis, wound healing, immune defense systems, and the production of particular neurotransmitters like collagen.

food sources: potatoes, broccoli, Brussels sprouts, cabbage, cauliflower, strawberries, melons, tomatoes, red and green peppers, and oranges.

Vitamin A

has a favorable impact on cancer cells and an anti-aging effect on the skin.

Food sources include liver, bell peppers, apricots, broccoli, bell peppers, sweet potatoes, spinach, cantaloupe, mango, and winter squash.

Vitamin E

has anti-inflammatory qualities and has been linked to slower cognitive decline in both elderly people and those with Alzheimer's disease.

Nuts, seeds, avocados, cereals, spinach, asparagus, broccoli, lettuce, onions, and fortified cereals are examples of food sources.

vitamins K

a crucial function in the transfer of calcium and the maintenance of bone density

Eggs, meat, tuna, kiwis, avocados, rhubarb, kale, broccoli, spinach, and asparagus are examples of food supplies.

Intake Of Protein

important to avoid muscle loss from sarcopenia.

sources of food include tofu, veggie burgers, chickpea beans, eggs, egg whites, fish, poultry, pork, and turkey.

Fiber

Poor nutritional intake, dehydration, or medication use all contribute to constipation in the elderly. Poorer quality of life, OCD, anxiety, paranoid thoughts, depression, and psychosis are Constipation.

Oatmeal, fruits (apples, berries, pears), vegetables, beans, and whole grains are all good sources of fiber.

Water hydration

Water hydration is crucial because being under hydrated can have a number of negative effects on health, including constipation. Remember that anything that contains caffeine causes you to lose water and acts as a diuretic.

Healthy Eating and Aging

As you age, it becomes even more crucial to maintain a balanced diet and eat healthily. Making sure you eat healthily is a terrific approach to ensure that you feel and look your best.

The Ideal Diet For Elderly People

Our bodies ability to age is greatly influenced by our diet. A diet high in nutrients and low in processed foods can help us feel young for longer by slowing down the aging process. Leafy greens, berries, seafood, nuts, and seeds are some of the greatest meals for anti-aging. Additionally, taking specific vitamins and supplements might offer extra advantages including lowering inflammation and illness prevention.

We are aware that it is never too late to make changes to support healthy aging since we know that good nutrition throughout the lifespan helps prevent chronic disease. Age-related changes in muscle and bone mass, such as osteoporosis, put older persons at higher risk for developing chronic diseases including cancer and heart disease. The good news is that by consuming nutrient-dense meals and having an active lifestyle, these people can reduce some of these risks.

Older persons frequently have fewer caloric needs than younger adults, but equal to or higher nutritional needs. This is frequently brought on by decreased exercise, modifications in metabolism, or age-related loss of bone and muscle mass. Chronic medical disorders, the consumption of several medications, and modifications in body composition all have an impact on the nutritional requirements of this population. Making every bite count and maintaining a nutritious diet is thus especially crucial for this age group.

The things we eat can significantly affect our fitness and quality of life., beauty, and risk of disease as we age. Our systems require a variety of nutrients to maintain the aging process and Some nutrients, like those that support good skin, may help halt the aging process.

It's important to realize that aging appropriately involves more than just nutrition and that eating certain meals won't make you seem notably younger.

Even so, incorporating nutrient-rich foods into your diet will help you age gracefully and feel your
best. Try to eat generally:

- healthful protein sources
- wholesome fats
- foods with lots of antioxidants

Here are some nutritious foods that promote good aging:

Extra virgin olive oil

Extra virgin olive oil is among the world's healthiest oils. It has a lot of healthy fats and antioxidants that support the body's defenses against inflammation and oxidative damage caused by an imbalance of free radicals.

Olive oil consumption has been associated with a reduced risk of several chronic illnesses, including Heart disease, metabolic syndrome, type 2 diabetes, and certain cancer types

Particularly, roughly 73% of olive oil is made up of monounsaturated fats (MUFAs). Because of this, a diet rich in MUFAs may reduce the aging process of the skin. of their potent anti-inflammatory properties.

Extra virgin olive oil is not only abundant in antioxidants like tocopherols and beta carotene, but it also has phenolic compounds with anti-inflammatory properties.

Extra virgin olive oil that has been cold-pressed is best since it is less processed and higher in antioxidants than oil that has been extracted in another way. Toss it in a salad or dip, it if you can.

The strong anti-inflammatory effects of olive oil may offer defense against chronic illness and rapid aging of the skin.

Green Tea

Green tea has strong antioxidants that can help the body fight off free radicals. Unstable molecules called free radicals are a consequence of how cells normally operate. They might grow in response to environmental conditions such as ultraviolet (UV) radiation or tobacco smoke. Free radicals can damage your cells if there are too many of them.

Antioxidants are useful in this situation. These compounds stabilize free radicals, protecting them from damage. Antioxidants are typically obtained from food, such as green tea.

Polyphenol-based antioxidants are particularly abundant in green tea. In particular, it contains a lot of gallic acids, catechins, and epigallocatechin gallate (EGCG).

These could lessen your danger of heart condition, cognitive decline, accelerated aging, and other chronic illnesses

By scavenging free radicals before they cause skin damage, the polyphenols present in green tea may help lessen external skin aging, which is brought on by environmental stressors like the sun and pollution.

Because of its antioxidant and anti-aging characteristics, green tea extract is actually used in many skin care products. Before green tea products can be suggested to slow down the aging process of the skin, more research is necessary. Having said that, eating a diet rich in antioxidants is linked to healthier skin and a lower risk of chronic disease. Additionally, adding more green tea to your diet will help you increase your intake of antioxidants.

Strong antioxidant capabilities are seen in green tea. As a result, it might aid in defending your skin against damage brought on by free radicals that might come from exposure to sunlight or other environmental causes.

Fatty Fish

Consuming fatty fish can aid in maintaining healthy skin. Its long-chain omega-3 fats are effective in reducing inflammation, heart disease, and other problems.

Additionally, studies have demonstrated that omega-3 fatty acids are connected to a robust skin barrier and may aid in reducing inflammation that harms the skin.

Salmon, one of the most popular fatty fish species, has extra advantages that can improve the condition of your skin.

First off, it includes astaxanthin, a carotenoid antioxidant that gives salmon its pink hue.

The high protein content of salmon and other fatty fish is crucial to consume in order for your body to manufacture collagen and elastin. The strength, fullness, and elasticity of the skin are due to these two molecules. Protein consumption helps wounds heal faster.

Lastly, fish has a lot of selenium. This mineral and antioxidant aids in DNA synthesis and repair, which may lessen and prevent UV-induced skin damage. Adequate amounts in the body may lessen how severe skin conditions like psoriasis are.

Salmon and other fatty fish are rich in protein, selenium, astaxanthin, and omega-3 fatty acids, all of which are linked to healthy skin.

Cocoa Or Dark Chocolate

The body's antioxidants, known as polyphenols, are widely present in dark chocolate.

It contains flavanols in particular, which have been connected to several health benefits, such as a reduced risk of cardiovascular disease, type 2 diabetes, and mental deterioration. Furthermore, it is believed that consuming a diet high in flavanols and other antioxidants can help shield the skin from UV damage and slow down the aging process.

Keep in mind that flavanol content increases with increasing cocoa content. Choose a type of dark chocolate that has at least 70% cocoa solids and low added sugar if you wish to include it in your diet.

Flavanols included in dark chocolate function as antioxidants in the body.

Vegetables

Antioxidants found in vegetables can help shield your skin from UV damage and support healthy skin renewal. The majority of veggies are low in calories and very nutrient-dense.

Antioxidants included in them can lower the risk of heart disease, cataracts, and several malignancies.

Also abundant in carotenoids like beta-carotene and lycopene are vegetables. According to some studies, eating a diet rich in carotenoids may shield the skin from the sun's UV rays, which are the principal cause of early aging of the skin. Several of the top sources of beta-carotene include: sweet potatoes, pumpkin, and carrots

Additionally, a lot of vegetables are high in vitamin C, a powerful antioxidant. Additionally, vitamin C is necessary for the production of collagen. The skin's primary structural component is collagen, but after the age of 25, the production of collagen starts to wane.

The vegetables with the highest vitamin C content are bell peppers, tomatoes, broccoli, and leafy greens.

Eating colorful veggies is crucial since each color signifies a different type of antioxidant that is good for your skin and general health.

At every meal, try to include two veggies, and always use sunscreen to protect your skin.

Flax Seeds

Flax seeds provide remarkable health advantages. They include lignans, a type of polyphenol that has antioxidant properties and may reduce your risk of contracting a chronic illness like breast cancer and heart disease.

They are also a good source of omega-3 fatty acid alpha-linolenic acid (ALA). An omega-3-rich diet supports a healthy skin membrane by promoting the hydration and plumpness of your skin.

Lignans are a class of antioxidants found in flaxseeds that aid in the body's defense against free radicals. Alpha-linolenic acid (ALA), an omega-3 that supports a healthy skin membrane, is also abundant in them.

Pomegranates

Pomegranates, like most fruits, are packed with beneficial elements. They include significant amounts of fiber, potassium, and vitamin K, all of which improve heart health. They are also abundant in antioxidants such as lignans, flavonols, tannins, and phenolic acids.

The antioxidants in pomegranates may also support healthy skin aging by reducing UV skin damage and brown spots brought on by sun exposure, according to several human and animal research.

Additionally, these antioxidants support the skin's ability to produce new collagen and protect the skin's existing collagen.

Pomegranate seeds and juice are an easy and wholesome way to add antioxidants to your diet.

Antioxidants found in abundance in pomegranates may aid in skin regeneration and shield the skin from sun-related damage.

Avocados

Avocados are a great source of fiber, heart-healthy fats, and a number of vital vitamins and minerals.

By supporting a healthy skin membrane, their high monounsaturated fat content may support the promotion of healthy skin, and their high antioxidant content may combat free radicals that harm and age the skin.

Avocados are a great method to add extra nourishment for good skin to your diet because of their excellent flavor and adaptability.

Tomatoes

Several of the remarkable health advantages that tomatoes offer can be due to their high lycopene content. The pigment lycopene is what gives tomatoes their red color. Additionally, it functions as an antioxidant to lower the risk of chronic illness.

Lycopene absorption from tomatoes is greatly increased when they are combined with healthy fats like avocado or olive oil. Lycopene, which is abundant in tomatoes and may offer some protection from the sun's UV radiation.

Collagen Peptides

The protein that is found in the body the most is collagen. For example, the skin and joints contain significant amounts of it. Our body starts to degrade collagen as we get older and generates it less efficiently. This may result in skin aging symptoms including wrinkles and drooping skin over time.

Consuming foods that promote collagen production will help you maintain the health of your skin for a longer period of time even though this process is unavoidable and a normal aspect of aging. Among these are foods high in protein and vitamin C. Avoiding actions that hasten collagen deterioration can also be beneficial. These include sunbathing in the sun and smoking cigarettes.

Consuming hydrolyzed collagen peptides, a smaller form of collagen that your body absorbs much more effectively may also help to reduce wrinkles and increase skin suppleness, hydration, and firmness. Eating a diet high in protein is essential for having good skin. If you want to increase your consumption of collagen even more, concentrate on consuming a diet high in protein. A few good sources of protein to consume consistently are: chicken, Fish, eggs Consuming collagen peptides that have been hydrolyzed enhances skin hydration, elasticity, and firmness.

Chapter 2

Exercise and Physical Activity

One of the best things we can do as we age is an exercise to keep our health and vigor. Regular exercise can lower the chance of developing chronic diseases like diabetes and heart disease, enhance cardiovascular health, and preserve muscle mass. However, it's crucial that older adults create an activity plan that is suitable for their level of fitness and physical capabilities. Walking, swimming, and low-impact aerobics are some examples of exercises that are appropriate for older persons.

Exercise for Older Adults:

To retain their independence and health, older adults must engage in physical activity and exercise. Despite the many advantages of physical activity, many older adults remain sedentary and don't work out frequently. This is because of a number of factors, including a reduction in physical function, ongoing medical issues, and a lack of enthusiasm. For older persons, regular physical activity has many health advantages, such as lowering the risk of chronic diseases, enhancing mobility, and maintaining independence. Exercise can also strengthen bones, lower the chance of falling, and enhance cardiovascular health. Furthermore, exercise can lower the incidence of depression and cognitive impairment.

The recommended minimum amount of daily moderate-intensity physical activity for older persons is 30 minutes. This can involve ordinary household tasks like cleaning or gardening as well as sports like walking, cycling, and swimming. Maintaining bone density and muscle strength can also be aided by resistance training, such as weightlifting.

Before beginning an exercise program, older persons should speak with their doctor, especially if they have any underlying medical issues. The intensity and length of their physical exercise can be gradually increased as older persons get more comfortable.

The advantages of routine exercise

For older persons, regular exercise has many advantages that can enhance their independence, independence level, and quality of life. Exercise can lower the chance of developing chronic diseases, improve mobility, and help maintain or even improve physical and mental health. Regular exercise might be essential to preserving general health and well-being when the body and mind deteriorate.

The enhancement of cardiovascular health for older persons is one of the most important advantages of regular exercise. Regular exercise can enhance heart health, lessen the risk of heart disease, and lower blood pressure. Exercise can also aid in boosting muscle strength and flexibility, which lowers the chance of falls and other accidents. This is crucial for older persons, who are more likely to fall and sustain injuries as their mobility and strength deteriorate.

Regular exercise helps lower the risk of developing chronic conditions like type 2 diabetes, obesity, and arthritis. Exercise has been demonstrated to help lower inflammation in the body, boost metabolism, and enhance insulin sensitivity. Additionally, physical exercise might enhance immune system performance, lowering the likelihood of contracting diseases and infections.

Another important advantage of regular exercise for older persons is improved mental health. Regular exercise has been demonstrated to enhance mood, lessen the signs of anxiety and depression, and enhance cognitive performance. Additionally, exercise can aid older persons' cognitive function, memory, and risk of dementia.

Long-term fitness and health benefits happiness and quality of life. We'll look at the real advantages of moving more.

1. The greatest advantage of exercising as you become older may be that it keeps you capable of living independently. Many elderly persons would want to live independently in their own homes for as long as possible, even though care homes are necessary for some. It's crucial to keep up an exercise routine that supports this way of life.

2. Improved cardiovascular health - Adults and older adults who engage in physical activity reduce their risk of cardiovascular disease by 35%. Stroke and heart attacks are medical conditions that, if they are not fatal, frequently have high-reaching effects.

3. May improve cognitive function - According to the Alzheimer's Society, over 1 million older adults

are expected to have dementia by 2025. Dementia affects many of these individuals. Exercise may be a strategy to lower the prevalence of the disease, according to certain studies.

4. Decreases anxiety and depression - Many elderly people may experience social isolation, disease, or disability, all of which can lead to mental health problems. Exercise has a number of cognitive advantages, including studies demonstrating a decrease in anxiety and sadness as well as a notable decrease in relapse when compared to other therapies.

5. Promotes flexibility - Joints and muscles become tight and immobile as a result of osteoarthritis pain, which is a major problem for elderly people. Even though age-related joint changes cannot completely be reversed with exercise, keeping your muscles and joints mobile is crucial for reducing pain.

6. Increases strength - Without exercise, muscles atrophy away. Similar to how exercise increases flexibility, the correct resistance training helps you maintain your independence by strengthening key muscle groups. This is especially helpful when standing up from a seated position, climbing and descending stairs, or when walking.

7. Increases bone density - Osteoporosis, a disorder that affects many elderly persons, causes the bones to deteriorate and become more prone to breaking. It has been demonstrated that regular resistance training helps keep bones strong as we age.

8. Prevents falls - People who lose their flexibility, strength, and coordination are at a higher risk of falling. Illness or disability may also be additional risk factors. The risk of slips, trips, and potential hospital admissions can be decreased by exercise.

9. Maintains hobbies - Losing the ability to engage in activities as a result of inactivity can have detrimental health and psychological effects. To be socially connected and active in life, one needs hobbies.

10. Aids in weight loss - Diet and inactivity can lead to weight gain as we age, which increases the prevalence of related medical diseases. Exercise might motivate you to follow a healthy diet in addition to burning calories. Additionally, engaging in physical activity can cut the risk of Type 2 diabetes by up to 40%.

11. Exercise is a habit that behavioral scientists have shown to help other beneficial routines,
like healthy eating and social engagement, by forming a foundational habit. Therefore, engaging in

physical activity can have a variety of beneficial side effects.

12. Enhances sleep - It has been shown that getting enough sleep can lower the risk of developing long-term physical and mental health issues, which makes it crucial for our emotional well-being. Exercise can promote physical and mental exhaustion, which can aid with sleep patterns.

13. Maintains social relationships - Exercising in a group setting not only holds you accountable but is also incredibly satisfying. Reinforcing social ties is essential to maintaining good health in later years, whether that be through a regular walk in the park with a buddy or an exercise class at the neighborhood recreation center.

14. Boosts confidence - Regular movement and training can enhance confidence in addition to the physical benefits, strengthening the mind-body link. Additionally, improving one's self-esteem through exercise might promote happiness and improve one's quality of life in later years.

15. Extends longevity - Research has shown that regular exercise can extend life expectancy by 3-5 years. Exercise not only extends life but also enhances its quality.

Even though it could be challenging to start exercising again after a long break, you'll soon get used to the development as your mobility and fitness levels rise.

It is essential to speak with your doctor or physiotherapist before working out if you have a medical problem or are unclear about what kind of physical exercise is suitable.

Additionally, it's wise to begin slowly and give your body time to adjust to a new level of activity in order to avoid damage.

How to create a productive fitness program

One of the best things you can do for your health is to start a workout regimen. Exercise can help you lose weight, increase your balance and coordination, lower your risk of developing chronic diseases, and even enhance your sleep patterns and sense of self-worth. There is additional good news. A fitness program can be initiated in only five simple steps.

1. **Determine your level of fitness**

You undoubtedly have a general concept of how you fit. However, calculating and documenting your baseline fitness scores might provide you with standards by which to compare your development.

Consider recording: To evaluate your flexibility, physical strength, and body composition:

your heart rate before and right away following a mile of walking (1.6 kilometers)

How long a mile of running takes, how long a mile of walking takes (2.41 kilometers)

How many pushups, either regular or modified, you can perform at once

How far you can stretch your legs out in front of you when seated on the floor?

your waist's measurement at the top of your hips

The BMI you're at

2. Create your exercise plan

It's simple to state that you'll work out each day. You'll need a plan, though. Keep the following in mind when you create your training program:

Think about your fitness targets. Are you beginning a workout regimen to aid with weight loss?

Or do you have another driving force, like training for a marathon? Having specific objectives might help you monitor your progress and stay motivated.

Make a regimen that is balanced. Get 75 minutes of severe aerobic exercise, 150 minutes of moderate aerobic exercise, or a combination of the two per week. The instructions advise spreading out this activity over the course of a week. At least 300 minutes per week are advised to provide even greater health benefits and help with weight loss or maintaining weight loss.

But even a little bit of exercise is beneficial. Even little bouts of activity spread out throughout the day can be beneficial to your health.

At least twice a week, perform a strength-training exercise for all the major muscle groups.

Start small and move slowly. When you first start exercising, proceed carefully and with caution. Consult your doctor or an exercise therapist for assistance in creating a fitness regimen that progressively increases your range of motion, strength, and endurance if you have an injury or a medical condition.

Include exercise in your everyday regimen. Finding the time to work out might be difficult. Make it simpler by scheduling exercise time just like you would any other appointment. Plan to read while riding a stationary bike, watch your favorite show while walking on the treadmill, or take a break to go for a stroll at work.

Consider including a variety of activities. Cross-training helps prevent exercise boredom by mixing up your workouts. Using low-impact exercises like a bike or water exercise as cross-training decreases your risk of overusing a particular muscle or joint or getting injured. Consider alternating between exercises that target various body areas, such as walking, swimming, and strength training.

Consider engaging in high-interval training. You engage in brief bursts of high-intensity exercise during high-interval intensity training, followed by recovery intervals of low-intensity exercise.

Allocate time for rest. Many people begin working out with an excessive amount of passion, working out for too long or too hard, and then giving up when their muscles and joints start to hurt or feel sore. Schedule recovery and rest periods for your body in between workouts.

Put it in writing. Having a documented plan in place could help you stay motivated.

3. Put your equipment together.

Most likely, you'll begin with athletic shoes. Choose footwear specifically made for the activity you have in mind. For instance, cross-training shoes are more supportive but weigh less than running shoes.

If you're going to spend money on exercise equipment, get something that will be useful, fun, and simple to use. Before buying your own equipment, you might wish to test out specific types at a fitness facility.

You might think about using fitness applications for smart devices or other activity-tracking gadgets, such as ones that can monitor your heart rate, measure your heart rate, and track your distance traveled.

4. Start out

You can now take action. Keep these suggestions in mind when your workout regimen gets started:

Start out slowly and progressively increase. Give yourself plenty of time to stretch or take a leisurely stroll to warm up and cool down. Then pick up the pace until you can maintain it for five to ten minutes without becoming too exhausted. Increase your exercise time progressively as your endurance gets better. Work your way up to exercising for 30 to 60 minutes most days of the week.

Break things up if necessary. You can spread out your workout throughout the day; you don't have to do it all at once. There are also aerobic advantages to shorter but more frequent sessions. A few quick workouts throughout the day may fit into your schedule more conveniently than a single 30-minute workout. Anything you do is preferable to doing nothing at all.

Be innovative. Perhaps you mix up your fitness routine with different exercises like walking, cycling, or rowing. Don't stop there though. Spend a night ballroom dancing or go on a weekend walk with your family. Find enjoyable activities to incorporate into your training regimen.

Be aware of your body. Take a break if you experience discomfort, breathlessness, vertigo, or nausea. You might be exerting too much effort.

Be adaptable. Give yourself permission to take a day or two off if you're not feeling well.

5. Track your development

Six weeks after you begin your program, and then every few months after that, retake your personal fitness evaluation. You might discover that in order to keep getting better, you need to work out for a longer period of time. Or, you might be pleasantly delighted to see that your level of exercise is just what you need to achieve your fitness objectives.

If your motivation wanes, try a different activity or make new goals. Additionally, working out with a friend or enrolling in a class at a gym might be beneficial.

Starting a fitness regimen is a crucial choice. However, it doesn't have to be onerous. You can create a lifelong healthy habit by properly planning and taking it slow.

Exercise and activities for older adults

Activity programs for older individuals should ideally combine aerobic exercise with strength/resistance training, flexibility exercises, and stretching. For the majority of older persons, trendy fitness regimens and high-intensity exercises are neither realistic nor safe. Here are some excellent exercises you may do to increase your strength, balance, and coordination while also increasing your mobility.

Yoga: Yoga is an easy exercise that won't put stress on your joints. Additionally, it aids with bone strength, core stability, flexibility improvement, and muscle development. To learn the fundamental positions, look for an introductory yoga class in your neighborhood. There are several yoga programs that are specially made for older persons and have alternatives for sitting and standing.

Pilates: Like yoga, Pilates is a moderate kind of exercise that is still effective. It focuses on developing a strong core to enhance balance and stability and has been shown to lessen the symptoms of Parkinson's, MS, and arthritis. The majority of the workouts are done while sitting or lying down. If it has been a while since you last exercised, Pilates is a good alternative to start.

Aerobic exercise: Including endurance exercise in your daily routine can assist enhance stamina on a daily basis, strengthen the lungs and airways, and promote cardiovascular health. What is an aerobic workout? For elderly people, walking, swimming, and riding a stationary bike are all beneficial activities. The suggested amount is 30 minutes per day. This may involve three

brief sessions of 10 minutes each scattered throughout the day.

No, bench pressing a hundred pounds counts as strength training! You may perform easy, low-impact bodyweight workouts at home to help you lose weight and build muscle. These include single-leg stands, squats, stair climbs, and wall push ups. Some strength-training exercises also include the use of resistance bands or small hand weights (between 1 and 2 pounds). For the best results, aim for two to three sessions per week.

One of the most crucial things you can do for your health as an older adult is to engage in regular physical activity. Some of the health advantages of exercise include less pain, improved mood, and a decreased chance of numerous diseases. It can improve your daily life, making it simpler to:

Perform errands and shop for daily necessities.

As you age, maintain your independence.

How many exercises Do older adults Need?

Throughout the day, concentrate on getting up and moving about more. Always know that any action is preferable to none. Before beginning a regimen of physical activity, see your doctor. You can adhere to these suggestions if you are 65 years of age or older, usually healthy, and free from any health restrictions:

At least 150 minutes a week should be spent engaging in moderate-intensity exercises, such as brisk walking or anything else that increases heart rate.

muscle-building exercise at least two days a week Include balance-enhancing stretches and exercises like standing on one leg.

Ready to Exercise More Regularly?

Increase your physical activity levels and intensity gradually as you go along. When increasing physical activity, consider your age, degree of fitness, and experience to help lower the chance of injury. Focusing on a low- to moderate-intensity activity, such as walking for 5–15 minutes per session, 2-3 times per week, is the ideal approach to get started. Walking has a low risk of injury and no known risk of serious cardiac events, according to research.

Chapter 3

Mental Health and Well-Being

When it comes to aging, mental health, and well-being are equally crucial to physical health. Older persons can retain a good attitude on life and increase general well-being by managing stress and depression, maintaining cognitive function, and participating in social activities. This chapter will discuss methods for preserving cognitive function, such as participating in mentally stimulating activities, as well as methods for coping with stress and sadness, such as mindfulness and meditation.

The link between mental health and aging

older adults frequently experience mental health issues, which can include isolation, anxiety and affective disorders, dementia, and psychosis, among other things. In addition, many elderly people experience sleep and behavioral issues, cognitive decline, or moments of bewilderment as a result of physical conditions or surgical procedures. The most prevalent mental health issues in older persons are anxiety or mood disorders,

particularly depression, which affects up to one in five of them. These mental health problems

typically respond favorably to treatment. Sadly, too many older adults do not ask for or receive the assistance they require. Mental health conditions that go undiagnosed and untreated can have devastating effects on older people and the people they care about.

Older Adults and Cognitive Health

The ability to think effectively, learn new things, and recall things is a crucial part of carrying out daily tasks. One facet of overall brain health is cognitive health.

What Is a Healthy Brain?

The term "brain health" describes how well a person's brain performs overall. The following are elements of brain health:

How well you think, learn, and remember is called cognitive health.

Your ability to make and control motions, including balance, is known as motor function.

How well you comprehend and react to emotions is known as emotional function (both pleasant and unpleasant)

How well you perceive and react to touch-related sensations like pressure, pain, and warmth is known as tactile function.

Age-related changes in the brain, injuries like strokes or traumatic brain injuries, mood disorders like depression, substance use disorders like addiction, and diseases like Alzheimer's disease can all have an impact on brain health. While there are some things that cannot be changed that affect brain health, there are many lifestyle adjustments that could have an impact.

The following actions may be related to cognitive health, according to a growing corpus of scientific study. Little adjustments can develop over time: Including these in your regimen might improve your performance.

Taking Good Care of Your Body

Maintaining good physical health may benefit mental wellness. One can:

*Obtain the suggested health examinations.

*Control long-term health issues like diabetes, hypertension, depression, and high cholesterol.

*Ask your doctor about the medications you use and any potential negative effects on your memory, sleep, and brain function.

*Reduce the chance of suffering a brain injury from falls or other mishaps.

*Limit your alcohol consumption (some medicines can be dangerous when mixed with alcohol).

*If you currently smoke, give it up. Avoid using chewing tobacco and other items with nicotine as well.

*Get enough sleep every night, ideally seven to eight hours.

*Reduce blood pressure

In addition to benefiting your heart, preventing or managing high blood pressure may also benefit your brain. High blood pressure raises the possibility of cognitive deterioration in old age.

There are many times no outward symptoms of sickness associated with high blood pressure. Even if you feel fine, regular medical visits can help detect changes in your blood pressure. Your doctor may advise exercise, dietary modifications, and, if necessary, medication to control or lower high blood pressure. These actions can aid in heart and brain health preservation.

Consume Healthy Foods

A nutritious diet can lower the chance of developing several chronic illnesses, such as diabetes or heart disease. It might also promote the health of your brain. Asian and Indian ladies laugh together

Fruits and vegetables, whole grains, lean meats, fish, and poultry, as well as low-fat or nonfat

dairy products, make up the bulk of a healthy diet. Salt, sugar, and solid fats should all be in moderation. Control your portion sizes and make sure you're getting enough water and other fluids.

Be Active Physically

Physical activity has various advantages, whether it be through routine exercise, housework, or other activities. It can assist you in:

*Maintain and develop your strength.

*Increase your energy and balance

*Prevent or postpone diabetes, heart disease, and other issues

*Boost your disposition and fight depression

Although a conclusive link between regular physical exercise and the prevention of Alzheimer's disease has not yet been established, studies correlate regular physical activity with advantages for the brain and cognition as well.

The ability of the human brain to preserve existing network connections and form new ones, both of which are crucial for cognitive health, was enhanced by exercise. Other research has demonstrated that exercise increases the size of a brain region crucial to memory and learning, improving spatial memory. Stretching and toning exercises that are not aerobic are regarded to be less beneficial to cognitive function than aerobic exercises like brisk walking. According to one study, the more time spent engaging in moderate physical activity, or how rapidly the brain converts glucose into fuel, the greater the increase in brain glucose metabolism, which may lower the chance of acquiring Alzheimer's disease.

Maintain Your Mind's Activity

The benefits of intellectual engagement on the brain may exist. People who participate in individually fulfilling activities, such as hobbies or volunteer work, report feeling happier and healthier. Developing new abilities may also help you think more clearly. For instance, research indicated that older persons who learned quilting or digital photography improved their memory more than those who merely engaged in social events or less mentally taxing pursuits. Some studies have shown the potential for enhancing the quality of life and well-being in older individuals by participation in arts such as music, theater, dance, and creative writing, from enhanced memory and self-esteem to lowered stress levels and greater social contact.

Your mind may stay engaged through a variety of activities. Read novels and magazines, for instance. Play video games. Attend or conduct a class. Develop a new hobby or talent. work or give back.

Maintain Relationships with Social Activities

Social interaction and community initiatives can help you feel less alone and more engaged with the world around you while also keeping your brain busy. Participating in social activities may increase well-being and reduce the risk of some health issues. People who participate in group activities that are both individually fulfilling and beneficial often live longer, are happier, and feel more purposeful. These activities appear to support the maintenance of their well-being and may enhance their cognitive function.

Visit your family and friends, then. Think about helping out a neighborhood organization or joining a group that shares your interests. Take part in a walking club with other older adults. Look into the senior center, area agency on aging, and other such programs in your neighborhood. More and more groups are meeting online as well, giving members a chance to interact from home with people who share their interests or seek assistance.

The ability of any of these measures to stop or slow down the onset of Alzheimer's disease and age-related cognitive decline is still unknown. However, some of these have been linked to a lower risk of dementia and cognitive impairment.

Control Your Stress

Life is certain to be stressful at times. Even short-term tension can help us concentrate and inspire us to act. Chronic stress, however, can alter the brain over time, impair memory, and raise the risk of Alzheimer's and other related dementias. There are various things you can do to assist manage stress and develop the capacity to recover from stressful events, including:

*Regular exercise Walking the outdoors or engaging in tai chi exercises can help you feel better.

*Create a journal entry. Writing down your ideas or concerns can assist you in letting go of a problem or discovering a fresh approach.

*Try some relaxation methods. Your body can unwind with the aid of techniques like mindfulness, which involves paying attention to the moment without passing judgment, or breathing exercises.

These can aid in lowering blood pressure, easing tension in the muscles, and lowering stress.

*Stay upbeat. Release resentments and things outside of your control, cultivate appreciation, or take a moment to appreciate the little things, such as the comfort of a cup of tea or the beauty of dawn.

Reduce the dangers to your cognitive health

It is believed that lifestyle, environmental, and genetic variables all affect cognitive health. Some of these elements may lead to a reduction in cognitive abilities and the capacity to carry out commonplace duties like driving, paying bills, taking medication, and cooking.

Genetic factors cannot be changed; they are passed down (inherited) from parent to kid. You can manage or adjust a lot of environmental and lifestyle factors, though, to lower your risk. These elements consist of:

- Some physical and mental health issues, such as hypertension or depression
- Injuries to the brain caused by falls or accidents
- Some medications, or the improper use of medications
- insufficient physical activity
- Dietary deficiencies

- Smoking
- Excessive alcohol consumption
- Sleep issues
- Loneliness and social isolation

Depression

Depression can affect anyone as they age, but there are ways to improve our moods and make our senior years healthy and happy.

Are you an older adult suffering from depression? Have you lost interest in the things you used to like? Do you experience feelings of hopelessness and helplessness? Is it becoming increasingly difficult for you to get through the day? you're not alone if this is the case. Depression can affect anyone as we age, regardless of our background or accomplishments. And the symptoms of elderly depression can have a negative impact on all aspects of your life, including your energy, appetite, sleep, and interest in work, hobbies, and relationships.

Unfortunately, far too many depressed older adults do not recognize the symptoms of depression or do not take the necessary steps to seek help. There are numerous reasons why elderly depression is frequently overlooked:

- You may believe you have a valid reason to be
- depressed or that depression is a natural part of aging.
- You may be isolated, which can lead to depression, with few people around to notice your distress.
- You may be unaware that your physical symptoms are symptoms of depression.
- You may be hesitant to express your feelings or seek assistance.

It's critical to understand that depression isn't a natural part of aging, nor is it a sign of weakness or character flaw. It can happen to anyone, at any age, regardless of background or previous achievements. While recent occurrences in your life as you get older, such as retirement, the death of loved ones, and declining health, can sometimes trigger depression, they don't have to keep you down. Whatever challenges you face as you age, there are steps you can take to reclaim your happiness and hope and enjoy your golden years.

Depression signs and symptoms in older adults

Recognizing depression in the elderly begins with an understanding of the signs and symptoms. Red flags for depression include:

- Feelings of sadness or despair.
- Aches and pains that are unexplained or exasperated.
- Loss of interest in social activities and hobbies.
- Loss of appetite or weight loss.
- Hopelessness or feeling helpless.
- Motivation and energy are lacking.
- Disruptions in sleep (difficulty falling asleep or staying asleep, oversleeping, or daytime sleepiness).
- Loss of self-esteem (worries about being a burden, feelings of worthlessness or self-loathing).
- Slow motion or speech.
- Increased consumption of alcohol or other drugs.
- Suicidal ideation stems from a fixation on death.
- Memory issues.
- Neglecting personal hygiene (skipping meals, forgetting meds, neglecting personal hygiene).

Managing Depression
Reach out and stay in touch.

Obtaining assistance is critical in overcoming depression. It can be difficult to maintain a healthy perspective and the effort required to overcome depression on your own. At the same time, the nature of depression makes seeking help difficult. When you're depressed, you tend to withdraw
and isolate, making it difficult to connect with even close family members and friends.

You may be too tired to talk, embarrassed about your situation, or guilty of ignoring certain relationships. But this is simply depression speaking. Keeping in touch with others and participating in social activities will improve your mood and outlook dramatically. Reaching out is not a sign of weakness, nor will it imply that you are a burden to others. Your loved ones genuinely care about you and want to assist you. And if you don't have anyone to turn to, it's never too late to make new friends and expand your support network.

Seek help from those who make you feel safe and cared for. The person with whom you speak does not need to be able to fix you; they simply need to

be a good listener—someone who will listen attentively
and compassionately without being distracted or judging you.

Make face-to-face time a priority. Phone calls, social media, and texting are excellent ways to stay in touch, but they cannot replace face-to-face quality time. The simple act of talking to someone face to face about how you feel can help to alleviate and prevent depression.

Even if you don't feel like it, try to keep up with social activities. When you're depressed, it's tempting to withdraw into your shell, but being around other people will make you feel less depressed.

Find ways to help others. It's nice to be supported, but research shows that providing support boosts your mood even more. So find ways to help others, both big and small: volunteer, be a listening ear for a friend, or do something nice for someone.

Take care of a pet. While nothing can replace a human connection, pets can bring joy and companionship into your life and make you feel less lonely. Caring for a pet can also get you out of your head and give you a sense of purpose, both of which are powerful antidepressants.

Do things that make you happy.

To overcome depression, you must engage in activities that both relax and energize you. Following a healthy lifestyle, learning how to better manage stress, setting limits on what you can do, and scheduling fun activities into your day are all part of this.

While you can't make yourself have fun or feel pleasure, you can force yourself to do things even when you don't want to. You may be surprised at how much better you feel once you're out in public. Even if your depression does not lift immediately, as you make time for enjoyable activities, you will gradually feel more upbeat and energetic.

Get better sleep

Aim for eight hours of sleep per night. Sleep problems are common in depression; whether you sleep too little or too much, your mood suffers. Learn healthy sleep habits to get on a better sleep schedule.

Maintain a healthy level of stress. Stress not only prolongs and worsens depression, but it can also precipitate it. Determine all of the stressors in your life, such as work overload, money problems, or unsupportive relationships, and devise strategies to relieve the pressure and regain control.

Use relaxation techniques. A daily relaxation practice can help alleviate depression symptoms, reduce stress, and increase feelings of joy and well-being. Yoga, deep breathing, progressive muscle relaxation, and meditation are all options.

Create a "wellness toolbox" to help you deal with depression. Make a list of things you can do to improve your mood quickly. The more "tools" you have for dealing with depression, the better. Even if you're feeling great, try to incorporate a few of these ideas into your daily routine.

Spend some time outside.

Make a list of the things you like about yourself.

Take some time to read a good book.

Watch a funny movie or television show.

Bathe in a long, hot bath.

Take care of a few minor details.

Play with your pet.

Talk to your friends and family in person.

Play some music.

Do something unexpected.

Get moving!

When you're depressed, even getting out of bed can be difficult, let alone working out! However, exercise is a powerful antidepressant and one of the most important tools in your recovery arsenal.

According to research, regular exercise can be just as effective as medication in alleviating depression symptoms. It also helps in the prevention of relapse once you've recovered.

Aim for at least 30 minutes of exercise per day to reap the most benefits. This does not have to be done all at once, and it is fine to start small. A 10-minute walk can lift your spirits for two hours. If you stick with it, your fatigue will improve. When you're depressed and exhausted, it can be difficult to begin exercising. However, studies show that if you stick to them, your energy levels will improve. Exercise will make you feel more energized and less fatigued, not the opposite.

Eat a healthy, anti-depression diet.

What you eat has a direct impact on how you feel. Reduce your consumption of foods that can have a negative impact on your brain and mood, such as caffeine, alcohol, trans fats, and foods high in chemical preservatives or hormones (such as certain meats)

Get your daily dose of sunlight.

Sunlight can help increase serotonin levels and boost your mood. Get outside during daylight hours whenever possible and expose yourself to the sun for at least 15 minutes per day. Remove your sunglasses (but never directly into the sun) and apply sunscreen as needed.

Confront negative thinking.

Do you ever feel powerless or weak? That bad things happen and you have little control over them? Is your situation hopeless? Depression has a negative impact on everything, including how you see yourself and your future expectations.

When these thoughts overwhelm you, remember that they are a symptom of your depression and that these irrational, pessimistic attitudes, known as cognitive distortions, are not realistic. When examined closely, they do not hold up. Even so, it can be difficult to give up. You won't be able to break free from this pessimistic mindset by telling yourself to "just think positive." It's often part of a lifelong pattern of thinking that's become so automatic that you're not even aware of it. The key is to recognize the negative thoughts that are fueling your depression and replace them with a more balanced way of thinking.

Stress

The body's response to physical or emotional demands is referred to as stress. Emotional stress can either cause or be a symptom of depression. A stressful situation can cause feelings of depression, which can make dealing with stress more difficult. High-stress events, such as job loss or the end of a long-term relationship, can result in depression. Not everyone who goes through these experiences becomes depressed. Biological factors may explain why one person experiencing a stressful situation develops depression while another does not.

Stress Management Suggestions

Stress management techniques can help you cope with depression. Stress reduction can prevent depressive symptoms. Some effective stress management techniques are as follows:

- obtaining adequate sleep
- consuming a nutritious diet
- exercising on a regular basis
- taking regular breaks from work or taking occasional vacations finding a relaxing hobby, such as gardening or woodworking consuming less caffeine or alcohol
- breathing exercises to reduce your heart rate

If your lifestyle choices are causing you stress, you may want to reconsider your approach to your personal or professional life. You can help reduce this type of stress by doing the following:

putting yourself under less pressure to perform at work or school, for example, by lowering your standards to a level you still find acceptable; not taking on as many responsibilities at work or activities at home; sharing responsibilities or delegating tasks to others around you; and surrounding yourself with supportive and positive friends and family members.

removing yourself from stressful situations or environments

Yoga, meditation, and attending religious services can also help you cope with stress. A combination of these methods could be even more effective. It is critical to discover what works best for you. And, no matter what you decide, having close friends and family members who are willing to support you is critical.

Speaking with a counselor, therapist, or other mental health professionals can also be beneficial in dealing with stress and depression. Talk therapy, alone or in combination with cognitive behavioral therapy (CBT) or medication, has been shown to be effective in treating depression and chronic stress.

Chapter 4

Social Connections and Support Systems

For aging adults, social connections and support systems are critical. Relationships with friends, family, and the community can help to improve overall well-being, reduce feelings of isolation and loneliness, and improve overall health. This chapter will look at how to establish and maintain relationships, as well as provide information on community resources and support groups that can be beneficial to older adults.

The significance of social connections for older adults

A Feeling Of Purpose

People who have spent years pursuing their careers or raising families may feel a loss of purpose after retirement. Being an active member of a social community can assist in meeting the need for belonging and meaning.

Improved Self-worth

Positive interaction with people of different ages on a regular basis may help to alleviate feelings of isolation. When older adults live in close quarters with others, they can experience a sense of self-worth and meaning, as well as find it easier to form peer relationships.

Improved Physical Health

When older adults are invited, accompanied, and encouraged to participate in physical activity, it can improve their physical well-being. Group exercise classes, for example, can help boost the immune system, reduce physical pain, and lower blood pressure. Even a short walk around the neighborhood to meet up with friends can help maintain physical fitness.

Improved Mental Health

older adults who are frequently lonely or isolated may suffer negative mental and physical consequences. older adults who are socially engaged on a regular basis, on the other hand, may be less likely to experience depression, stress, and anxiety.

Here are some suggestions for staying socially active and making new friends as you get older:

1. Become a volunteer

Volunteering is a fulfilling way to reconnect with old friends and make new ones. The maturity and life experience of mature volunteers are invaluable. It enables you to put your life skills to use and share them with others.

2. Participate

Participating in your community allows you to meet new people while doing what you enjoy.

Join a club or start your own, Join your local men's shed, Start a team sport or take regular exercise classes, Contribute to your local community garden, Attend local council meetings, If you live in a retirement village or receive home care, participate in community events or social outings organized by your provider.

3. Reconnect with old acquaintances

If starting new friendships from scratch feels too daunting, reach out to old friends with whom you've lost touch. When you reconnect with people you used to be close to, you can pick up
right where you left off.

4. Maintain consistency

Friendships, like any other type of relationship,

necessitate effort to maintain.

Set a weekly date with your friends to do something you all enjoy, such as going to the park, watching a football game, or watching movies. Having a set time each week increases your chances of catching up and spending time together, strengthening your friendship.

5. Alter your living circumstances

Changing your living situation is another way to combat loneliness. If you live alone, invite a friend to join you or advertise for a roommate.

6. Accept more opportunities

It may seem obvious, but saying yes more often when friends invite you out or when the family wants to catch up is a great way to meet new people. Going out to socialize with people you already feel comfortable with increases your chances of meeting new people.

Chapter 5

Chronic Disease Management

Chronic diseases such as diabetes, heart disease, and osteoarthritis are common as we age. Controlling these conditions can help to improve overall health and reduce the likelihood of complications.

Chronic diseases are defined broadly as conditions that last a year or more and necessitate ongoing medical attention, limit daily activities, or both.

Many chronic diseases are caused by a small number of risk factors:

Tobacco use and. Secondhand smoke exposure.

Poor nutrition, including a lack of fruits and vegetables and a high sodium and saturated fat intake.

Inactivity on the physical level.

Excessive alcohol consumption.

Common chronic conditions in the older adults

Chronic Obstructive pulmonary disease (COPD)

Chronic obstructive pulmonary disease (COPD), a chronic disease that includes two main conditions—emphysema and chronic bronchitis—was treated by 11% of older adults. COPD makes breathing difficult, causing shortness of breath, coughing, and chest tightness.

Quitting or avoiding smoking is the most effective way to prevent COPD or slow its progression. Avoid secondhand smoke, chemical fumes, and dust, all of which can irritate your lungs.

If you already have COPD, finish the treatments your doctor has prescribed, get the flu and pneumonia vaccines your doctor has recommended, and stay active.

Dementia and Alzheimer's disease

Eleven percent of Medicare-eligible older adults were treated for Alzheimer's disease or another form of dementia. Alzheimer's disease is a type of dementia that causes memory loss and difficulty thinking or problem-solving to the point where it interferes with daily activities. Dementia is not a normal part of aging, but rather the result of changes in the brain over time.

The most important risk factors for these chronic conditions are often beyond your control, such as age, family history, and genetics, but studies have shown that incorporating the following habits into your lifestyle can slow or prevent their onset.

Exercise. Staying active is beneficial not only to your heart but also to your brain.

Sleep. Because your brain works hard while you sleep, getting at least 7 hours of deep sleep per night is critical.

Be mindful of your diet. According to research, certain foods can have a negative impact on your brain.

Heart attack

Fourteen percent of older adults were treated for heart failure, a condition in which the heart is unable to adequately supply blood and oxygen to all of the body's organs. To meet the body's needs, the heart may enlarge, gain muscle mass, or pump faster, leaving you tired, light-headed, nauseous, confused, or lacking in appetite. The best way to reduce your risk of coronary heart disease and high blood pressure is to follow your doctor's recommendations.

Chronic kidney disease (CKD)

Eighteen percent of older adults were treated for chronic kidney disease (CKD), which is characterized by a gradual loss of kidney function over time. People with CKD are more likely to develop heart disease or kidney failure. To prevent or reduce CKD symptoms, you can do the following:

Learn what causes kidney damage. Diabetes and high blood pressure are the two most common risk factors for kidney damage, so preventing these diseases is your best bet.

Early detection and treatment are essential. Talk to your doctor on a regular basis, keep up with screenings, and fill any prescriptions you may require to alleviate symptoms.

Diabetes

Diabetes, which occurs when your body is resistant to or does not produce enough insulin, was treated by 27% of older adults. Insulin is the substance that your body uses to extract energy from food and distribute it to your cells. If this does not occur, you will develop high blood sugar, which can lead to complications such as kidney disease, heart disease, or blindness.

You may do the following to prevent or manage diabetes.

Eating a healthy diet, including tracking carbohydrate and calorie intake, and discussing alcohol consumption with your doctor.

Exercising for 30 minutes five times per week to keep blood glucose levels in check and weight gain under control.

If you have pre-diabetes, you can safely lose 5-7% of your body weight.

Heart ischemia (or coronary heart disease)

Twenty-nine percent of older adults were treated for ischemic heart disease, a condition caused by plaque buildup in the arteries leading to the heart. Atherosclerosis reduces the amount of oxygen-rich blood delivered to the heart. This can lead to complications such as blood clots, angina, or a heart attack.

You can help yourself by incorporating the following habits:

Limit your intake of sugar and salt, and avoid saturated and trans fats.

Each night, get seven to eight hours of sleep.

Maintain a healthy level of stress.

Perform regular cardio exercises.

Smoking should be avoided.

Discuss with your doctor the major risk factors, such as high cholesterol and high blood pressure.

Arthritis

Thirty-one percent of older adults received treatment for arthritis, a joint inflammation that causes pain and stiffness and is more common in women.

You can take the following steps to delay the onset of arthritis or manage its symptoms:

To improve function and reduce pain, exercise at least 5 times per week for 30 minutes each time. Include a variety of aerobic, strength-building, and stretching exercises.

Maintain a weight that is appropriate for your height—losing one pound can relieve four pounds of pressure on your knees.

Always keep your back, legs, and arms supported.

Avoid joint injuries by taking precautions.

Avoid smoking.

High cholesterol

High cholesterol was treated in 47 percent of older adults, a condition that occurs when your body has an excess of bad fats (or lipids), resulting in clogged arteries, which can lead to heart disease.

When it comes to preventing or managing high cholesterol, you can control the following lifestyle factors:

Smoking cessation and excessive alcohol consumption

Being physically active every day

Weight management

Reduce your intake of saturated and trans fats.

Hypertension (high blood pressure)

Fifty-eight percent of older adults were treated for hypertension, a common condition involving both the amount of blood your heart pumps and the resistance of your arteries to blood flow. High blood pressure, also known as hypertension, occurs when your heart pumps a lot of blood and you have narrow arteries that resist the flow. The danger of hypertension is not only that it can go undetected for years, but it can also lead to other serious health problems such as strokes and heart attacks.

You can try to prevent or reduce high blood pressure by doing the following:

Keeping a healthy weight. Even a ten-pound weight loss can lower blood pressure.

Control your stress levels

Limit your intake of salt and alcohol.

Check your blood pressure on a regular basis—the sooner you detect pre-hypertension, the better your chances of avoiding high blood pressure.

When these strategies fail to alleviate your chronic condition,

Chronic disease prevention

Some chronic diseases are unpreventable because they are inherited or the cause is unknown. Type 1 diabetes, multiple sclerosis, rheumatoid arthritis, and cystic fibrosis are a few examples.

Other chronic conditions can develop as a result of risk factors that people can control. Type 2 diabetes, kidney disease, certain lung diseases, and stroke are all examples.

You can reduce your risk of developing a preventable chronic condition by doing the following:

smoking cessation

sufficient physical activity

reducing your alcohol intake eating well\maintaining a healthy blood pressure\shaving good cholesterol levels.

Managing Chronic Conditions

Effective chronic condition management can help:

improve your overall health and happiness

avoid or postpone complications

slow your disease's progression

What can I do to improve my condition management?

Learn everything you can about your illness. Read widely, but be cautious: not everything you read is true.

Learning about your condition will allow you to take control of your health and select treatments that are right for you. It will also assist you in asking the appropriate questions of your doctor.

Actively managing your condition and assisting in the treatment of symptoms can improve your quality of life.

Which medical professionals can assist me in managing my chronic health condition?

If you have a chronic illness, having a team of health professionals involved in your care will most likely benefit you.

Make sure you have a doctor who understands you and your way of life. It will be much easier for you if you have one person who is central to your health care.

Request a Chronic Disease Management (CDM) plan from your doctor. These plans offer a systematic approach to managing your illness. They are mutually agreed upon by you and your doctor, and they include ongoing care from a team of health professionals.

Specialist physicians and allied health professionals

Other healthcare providers who may be involved in your care include specialists and allied health professionals. The following are examples.

Counseling and information about government and community support services can be provided by a social worker. Speak with your local community health center about how a social worker can assist you in managing your chronic condition.

A dietitian is a nutritionist who can provide expert nutrition and diet advice.

An occupational therapist can assist you in maintaining, regaining, or improving your independence.

If you are experiencing pain or difficulty moving, see a physiotherapist.

A psychologist to assist you in dealing with the difficulties of chronic illness.

How else can I assist in the management of my chronic condition?

A healthy lifestyle can assist you in managing your chronic condition. A healthy lifestyle includes the following elements:

A healthy diet, being as active as possible, getting enough sleep, not smoking, and limiting the amount of alcohol you consume Medicines

Understand your medications and take them exactly as directed.

If you are taking medications for an extended period of time, have your doctor review them on a regular basis to ensure they are still appropriate.

Chapter 6

Sleep and Aging

The significance of sleep for the elderly

Sleep is an essential mechanism for everyone, regardless of age. It has the ability to regenerate energy and heal both physical and mental damage. So, how will it benefit your loved ones in their golden years?

Sleep has numerous advantages for older people, including improved overall health and quality of life.

what exactly are sleep disorders?

Sleep disorders are conditions that interfere with or prevent you from getting enough restful sleep, resulting in daytime sleepiness and other symptoms. Everyone can have sleep problems from time to time. It's likely you have a sleep disorder if you have any of the following symptoms:

You frequently have trouble sleeping.

Even though you slept for at least seven hours the night before, you are frequently tired during the day.

You have a diminished or impaired ability to engage in regular daytime activities

Sleep disorders that are common and how to treat them

Insomnia

Insomnia is a sleep disorder in which people struggle to fall or stay asleep. Insomniacs exhibit one or more of the following symptoms:

Having trouble falling asleep.

Frequently waking up during the night and having Difficulty falling back asleep.

Getting out of bed too early.

Sleeping is not refreshing.

Having at least one daytime problem due to lack of sleep, such as fatigue, sleepiness, mood problems, concentration problems, accidents at work or while driving, etc.

Insomnia varies in duration and frequency of occurrence. About half of the adults have occasional bouts of insomnia, and one in ten has chronic insomnia. Insomnia can occur on its own or in conjunction with medical or psychiatric conditions. Insomnia can be temporary (acute or adjustment insomnia) or chronic (chronic insomnia). It can also come and go, with periods when a person does not have any sleep problems. Acute or adjustment insomnia can last anywhere from a single night to several weeks. Chronic insomnia occurs when a person experiences insomnia at least three nights per week for a month or longer.

Sleep Apnea

Sleep apnea is a potentially fatal sleep disorder in which a person's breathing is interrupted while sleeping. Not treated sleep apnea causes people to stop breathing repeatedly during the night.

Obstructive and central sleep apnea are the two types.

The more common condition is obstructive sleep apnea (OSA). It is caused by an obstruction of

the airway, which usually occurs when the soft tissue in the back of the throat collapses while sleeping. Snoring, daytime sleepiness, fatigue, restlessness during sleep, gasping for air while sleeping, and difficulty concentrating are all symptoms of OSA.

The airway is not blocked in central sleep apnea (CSA), but the brain fails to tell the body to breathe. Because it affects the function of the central nervous system, this type is known as central apnea. People with CSA may gasp for air, but the majority report frequent nighttime awakenings.

Restless Legs Syndrome
RLS is a sleep disorder characterized by an intense, often irresistible urge to move one's legs. This sensation is caused by resting, such as lying down in bed or sitting for extended periods of time, such as while driving or watching a movie. RLS is most common in the evening, making it difficult to fall and stay asleep. It has been due to issues with daytime sleepiness, irritability, and concentration. People suffering from RLS frequently want to walk around and shake their legs to help relieve the uncomfortable sensation.

Narcolepsy
Narcolepsy is a sleep-regulation disorder that affects the control of sleep and wakefulness. Narcolepsy causes excessive daytime sleepiness as well as intermittent, uncontrollable episodes of falling asleep during the day. These unexpected sleep attacks can happen at any time of day and during

any form of activity. Some narcolepsy patients do experience sudden muscle weakness in response to laughter or other emotions.

Treatment And Management

Healthcare providers recommend a variety of treatments, including:

Counseling: Cognitive behavior therapy is recommended by some sleep specialists. This particular counseling will help you to "recognize, challenge, and change stress-inducing thoughts" that can keep you awake at night.

Medications and nutritional supplements.

Maintaining a regular sleep schedule is an example of sleep hygiene.

Get some exercise on a regular basis.

Reduce the amount of noise.

Reduce the amount of light.

Adjust the temperature to your preference.

Your healthcare provider will make recommendations based on your specific situation.

Chapter 7

skin Care And Aging,

Aging's Effects On The Skin

As we age, our skin is subjected to a variety of forces, including the sun, harsh weather, and bad habits. We can, however, take steps to keep our skin supple and youthful.

Your lifestyle, diet, heredity, and other personal habits will all influence how your skin ages. For example, smoking can generate free radicals, which are once-healthy oxygen molecules that have become overactive and unstable. Free radicals damage cells, causing premature wrinkles among other things.

There are additional reasons. Normal aging, sun exposure (photoaging), pollution, and loss of subcutaneous support are the primary causes of wrinkled, spotted skin (fatty tissue between your skin and muscle). Stress, gravity, daily facial movement, obesity, and even sleep position are all factors that contribute to skin aging.

What Skin Changes Occur With Age?

Changes like these occur naturally as we age:

The skin roughens.

Lesions, such as benign tumors, can form on the skin.

Skin becomes saggy. With age, the skin loses its elastic tissue (elastin), causing it to hang loosely.

The skin becomes more translucent. This is caused by epidermis thinning (surface layer of the skin).

Skin becomes more delicate. This is caused by a flattening of the area where the epidermis and dermis (the skin layer beneath the epidermis) meet.

Skin becomes more prone to bruises. This is due to the fact that the blood vessel walls are thinner.

Changes beneath the skin become visible as we age. They are as follows:

Fat loss beneath the skin in the cheeks, temples, chin, nose, and eye area can cause a leaner appearance, loosening skin, sunken eyes, and a "skeletal" appearance.

After the age of 60, bone loss, particularly around the mouth and chin, can cause puckering of the skin around the mouth.

Drooping of the nasal tip and accentuation of the bony structures in the nose is caused by cartilage loss in the nose.

Maintaining Healthy skin as You Age

The sun contributes significantly to the premature aging of our skin. Some other things we do can expedite the aging of our skin. Dermatologists give the following advice to their patients to assist them in preventing premature skin aging.

*Every day, protect your skin from the sun. Sun protection is essential whether you're spending the day at the beach or running errands. Seek shade, wear sun-protective clothing, such as a lightweight and long-sleeved shirt, pants, a wide-brimmed hat, and UV-protective sunglasses, and apply sunscreen that is broad-spectrum, SPF 30 (or higher), and water-resistant. Every day, apply sunscreen to all exposed skin that is not covered by clothing. Look for clothing with an ultraviolet protection factor (UPF) label for better protection.

*Stop smoking if you do. Smoking precipitates the aging process of the skin. It is responsible for wrinkles and a dull, sallow complexion.

*Avoid making the same facial expressions over and over. When you make a facial expression, the underlying muscles contract. These lines become permanent if you repeatedly contract the same muscles over a long period of time. Squinting lines can be reduced by putting on sunglasses.

*Consume a nutritious, well-balanced diet. According to the findings of a few studies, eating plenty of fresh fruits and vegetables may help prevent damage that leads to premature skin aging. According to the findings of research studies, a diet high in sugar or other refined carbohydrates can hasten aging.

*Reduce your alcohol consumption. Alcohol is abrasive to the skin. It dehydrates the skin and eventually damages it. This may make us appear older.

*Exercise. A few studies have found that moderate exercise can improve circulation and boost the immune system. As a result, the skin may appear to be more youthful.

*Gently cleanse your skin. Scrubbing your skin can cause irritation. Irritating your skin hastens its aging. Gentle washing removes pollution, makeup, and other substances from your skin without irritating it. Wash your face at least twice a day and after heavy sweating. Perspiration irritates the skin, especially when wearing a hat or helmet, so you should wash your skin as soon as possible after sweating.

Common skin problems and how to treat them

Your skin changes as you get older. It thins out, loses fat, and no longer appears as plump and smooth as it was. Your veins and bones are more visible. Scratches, cuts, and bumps may require more time to heal. Years of suntanning or being out in the sun for an extended period of time can cause wrinkles, dryness, age spots, and even cancer. However, there are things you can do to protect your skin and improve its feel and appearance.

Here are eight skin conditions in elderly people, as well as what older people, loved ones, and caregivers should be aware of.

1. Bruising easily

Why do the elderly bruise so easily? Skin thins with age, and there is less fat to cushion it. Furthermore, blood vessels are more delicate and easily broken. Bruises are caused by blood leakage from blood vessels, so more broken vessels equal more bruising. People over the age of 65 who take blood thinners or even over-the-counter pain relievers like aspirin or ibuprofen may bruise more easily.

A minor bump or scrape can cause a surprising amount of bruising, leading concerned loved ones to wonder what's going on. The bruises are usually not harmful. However, anyone who develops large bruises on a regular basis with no logical explanation should see a doctor to rule out an underlying health problem.

Take action now

To treat bruises,

Apply a cold compress to the affected area for up to 20 minutes at a time.

Apply Dermaka cream, a bruise treatment made of plant extracts and vitamins, as directed on the package.

When resting, keep a bruised leg or foot elevated.

2. Itching and dryness

Dry skin in the elderly is very common; in fact, more than half of the elderly have it. One cause is the loss of sweat and oil glands. Another factor could be a lack of fluids. Furthermore, certain chronic health conditions, such as diabetes and kidney disease, as well as some of the medications used to treat them, can cause dryness and itching.

The skin may crack and become painful. Scratching can cause skin irritation and allow infection-causing germs to enter the body.

Take action now

If you have itchy, dry skin:

Use a moisturizing soap and take shorter, cooler baths or showers (skip the deodorant soap)

Use a moisturizing ointment or cream on a daily basis. (Avoid lotions, which are higher in water content.) CeraVe, Cetaphil, and Vanicream are all gentle, effective moisturizers.

Drink plenty of water.

If the air is dry, turn on a humidifier.

Inform your doctor if the itching persists. It could be an indication of a liver, kidney, or thyroid problem.

3. Age

As a result of years of sun exposure, the skin of older adults is frequently dotted with age spots. These flat, tanned, or dark brown spots, also known as liver spots, typically appear on sun-exposed skin, such as the face, arms, and back of the hands. They're not dangerous.

Take action now

Wear sunscreen with at least 30 SPF to help prevent the development of new age spots.

Consult a dermatologist to ensure that the spots are age spots and not something else, especially if their appearance changes.

A skin healthcare practitioner can treat age spots if they bother you.

4. Skin tags

Skin tags are soft, spongy, flesh-colored tissue growths that most commonly appear on the eyelids, neck, thighs, and skin folds such as the armpits, groin, and under the breasts. On small stalks, they may dangle from the skin. Skin tags are more common in women, overweight people, older people, and diabetics. They can become irritated if their clothing rubs against them or if their jewelry snags on them.

Take action now

Skin tags are not dangerous, but if you want one removed, consult a dermatologist. It will be removed by a dermatologist.

Do not try to remove a skin tag on your own. It's a bad idea for a number of reasons.

5. Shingles

Adults who had chickenpox as children are at risk of developing shingles. older adults are especially vulnerable.

Shingles are characterized by burning, itching, tingling, or extreme sensitivity in one area of the skin. A painful rash appears next, often accompanied by a fever or headache. The rash eventually develops into blisters. Complications such as skin infections and long-term nerve pain are possible.

Take action now

Consult a physician as soon as symptoms appear. Early treatment with oral antiviral medication has been shown to shorten the duration and severity of an outbreak.

Take an over-the-counter pain reliever and treat itching with cool compresses, calamine lotion, and lukewarm baths with colloidal oatmeal (oats ground into a fine powder).

Get both doses of the Shingrix vaccine to prevent shingles.

6. Pressure ulcers

Bedridden or wheelchair-bound elderly people are vulnerable to open wounds known as bed sores or pressure ulcers. These form in pressure points when sitting or lying down, such as the

tailbone, shoulder blades, backs of the knees, and heels. Diabetes, poor circulation, and poor

nutrition all increase the risk of bed sores.

Prevention is essential. Once formed, bed sores can be extremely difficult to treat and may become infected.

Take action now

Reposition yourself in bed every two hours. Change positions in a wheelchair every 15 minutes.

Maintain clean and dry skin.

Keep an eye out for redness and warmth in one area of the skin; this is an early warning sign. If you are a caregiver and notice this or a sore, scrape, or blister, call the doctor. To coordinate care, a wound care nurse may be required.

Consider a gel or foam mattress topper or alternating air pressure mattress to help prevent pressure sores.

7. Skin abrasions

The fragile skin of elderly adults tears more easily, especially if they take corticosteroids, which can weaken the skin. When you bump into something or when a caregiver removes wound tape or a dressing, the skin may tear.

Take action now

To keep skin hydrated and prevent tears, use moisturizer and drink plenty of water.

To protect your skin, wear long pants and a long-sleeved shirt or arm sleeves.

If a small tear occurs, clean the wound gently with soap and water. Replace the skin flap, if present, and then cover the wound with gauze.

Consult a doctor if you have more severe tears or notice signs of infection, such as redness, swelling, fever, worsening pain, or a foul odor.

8. Skin cancer

The sun is the leading cause of skin cancer. Skin cancer can also be caused by tanning beds and sunlamps. Skin cancer can affect anyone, regardless of skin color. People with fair skin who freckle easily are most vulnerable. Skin cancer can be cured if it is detected early enough before it spreads to other parts of the body.

Skin cancers are classified into three types. Basal cell carcinoma and squamous cell carcinoma are two types that grow slowly and rarely spread to other parts of the body. These cancers are typically found on areas of the skin that are frequently exposed to sunlight, such as the head, face, neck, hands, and arms. However, they can occur anywhere in your body. Melanoma is the third and most dangerous type of skin cancer. It is less common than the others, but it can spread to other organs and be fatal.

Take action now

Examine your skin once a month for any signs of cancer. Skin cancer is almost never painful. Look for changes such as a new growth, an unhealed sore, or a bleeding mole.

Examine moles, birthmarks, and other areas of the skin for "ABCDEs."

A = Asymmetry. One-half of the growth looks different from the other half

B = Borders that are erratic

C = Color changes or multiple colors

D = Diameter larger than that of a pencil eraser

E = Evolving, which refers to growth changes in size, shape, symptoms (itching, tenderness), surface (especially bleeding), or color shades.

If you notice any of these symptoms, see your doctor right away to rule out skin cancer.

Conclusion

Aging is a normal part of life, but with the right strategies, we can keep our health and vitality for many years. The key to staying active is to:

Eat a Balanced and Nutritious Diet: Eating a balanced and nutritious diet can help keep the body in good shape, delay the aging process, and promote healthy skin and hair.

Regular physical activity has been shown to improve both mental and physical health, resulting in a younger, more energetic appearance. Regular physical activity also benefits cardiovascular health, bone and muscle strength, and cognitive function.

Get Enough: Adequate sleep promotes physical and mental health, reduces stress, and improves overall well-being. Sleep deprivation can cause wrinkles, dark circles, and dull skin. A good night's sleep can help maintain youthful, refreshed, and radiant skin.

Stay Hydrated: Staying hydrated allows the body to perform at its best and promotes healthy skin, hair, and nails.

Tobacco and excessive alcohol consumption should be avoided because they can cause serious health problems and hasten the aging process.

Stress management: Chronic stress can cause the hormone cortisol to be produced, causing the body to age faster.

Stress management activities like meditation, yoga, and exercise can help reduce the negative effects of stress on the body and mind.

Reading, puzzles, or learning a new skill can help maintain cognitive function and delay the onset of age-related declines.

Building and maintaining strong social connections have been shown to improve mental and emotional well-being, reduce stress, and increase life satisfaction.

Use sunscreen, moisturize daily, and avoid harsh chemicals to keep your skin looking young and radiant.

Avoid Prolonged Sun Exposure: Prolonged sun exposure can cause skin damage, resulting in wrinkles, fine lines, and age spots. Additionally, avoiding excessive sun exposure and using sunscreen can help prevent skin damage and lower the risk of skin cancer.

Check-ups with a healthcare professional on a regular basis can help detect and prevent health problems early, improve overall health, and increase life expectancy.

staying young entails making healthy choices and taking care of your body. Regular exercise, healthy eating, adequate rest, and stress management can help you look and feel young and energetic. Taking care of your skin, limiting sun exposure, and staying hydrated are all essential steps in maintaining a youthful appearance.

Taking charge of your health and longevity is a proactive and empowering step toward living a longer, happier, and more fulfilling life. Making healthy lifestyle choices can improve not only the quantity but also the quality of your life. There are numerous strategies you can use to promote healthy aging, such as eating a well-balanced diet, getting regular exercise, managing stress, or engaging in mentally stimulating activities. So, instead of waiting until it's too late, take charge of your health and longevity today. Make an investment in yourself and your future. You will not only increase your chances of living a longer life, but also of living a life full of vitality, happiness, and purpose by doing so.